Sleeping Secrets

How to Get the Good Night Sleep You Deserve

By: Emil McAdams

9781681279602

Publishers Notes

Disclaimer – Speedy Publishing LLC

This publication is intended to provide helpful and informative material. It is not intended to diagnose, treat, cure, or prevent any health problem or condition, nor is intended to replace the advice of a physician. No action should be taken solely on the contents of this book. Always consult your physician or qualified health-care professional on any matters regarding your health and before adopting any suggestions in this book or drawing inferences from it.

The author and publisher specifically disclaim all responsibility for any liability, loss or risk, personal or otherwise, which is incurred as a consequence, directly or indirectly, from the use or application of any contents of this book.

Any and all product names referenced within this book are the trademarks of their respective owners. None of these owners have sponsored, authorized, endorsed, or approved this book.

Always read all information provided by the manufacturers' product labels before using their products. The author and publisher are not responsible for claims made by manufacturers.

This book was originally printed before 2015. This is an adapted reprint by Speedy Publishing LLC with newly updated content designed to help readers with much more accurate and timely information and data.

Speedy Publishing LLC

40 E Main Street, Newark, Delaware, 19711

Contact Us: 1-888-248-4521

Website: http://www.speedypublishing.co

REPRINTED Paperback Edition: 9781681279602

Manufactured in the United States of America

Dedication

I dedicate this book to my younger sisters Abigail and Aleah, who hated going to sleep when they were little girls now they cherish every hour of it.

Table of Contents

Chapter 1- The Basics of a Good Nightly Sleep

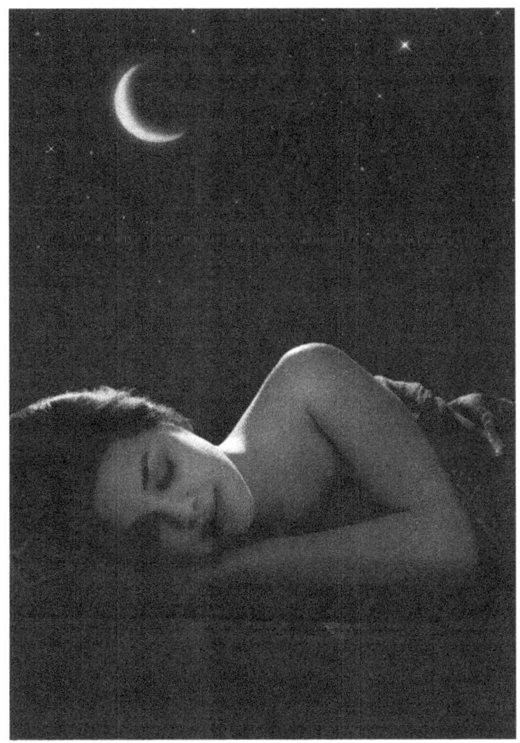

Sleep can help people fight the negative effects of stress and tiredness more effectively every day. It's something that alters the consciousness of an individual while resting during evening hours. This naturally recurring state allows the mental health and body of a person to be rejuvenated regularly every morning.

If people will never sleep regularly at night, their bodies will suffer from several kinds of serious medical conditions and diseases. Poor quality of sleep usually encourages the brain to release several kinds of harmful toxins in the different parts of a human body. These toxins allow a human body to suffer from cancer, heart diseases, obesity/overweight cases and other dangerous medical conditions that are not too easy to treat.

Sleeping Secrets

Poor quality of sleep can also make a person weak and irritated every day. It's one of the things that can make a person vulnerable to the negative effects of stress every day. An individual has to sleep for almost eight hours every night in order to experience all benefits that a rejuvenating sleep can provide.

There are so many things that can affect the ability of a person to achieve a good quality of sleep every night. One of these factors is an uncomfortable sleeping environment.

Those people who usually sleep in places that are always surrounded with light have uncomfortable sleeping environment. The same thing goes to those individuals whose bedrooms are not too far from public highways where several kinds of noises that can be produced by vehicles and pedestrians are always available. One of the most effective ways to have a good quality of nightly sleep is to prepare a safe and comfortable sleeping environment.

Look for a place that's always free and protected from noise pollution that can be produced by several kinds of environmental noises. Construct a bedroom in its area and provide its windows with wonderful curtains where sunlight can't enter during sunrise.

An excellent sleeping environment refers to a place that's totally inaccessible for all things that can disturb a person while sleeping like environment noises and light.

Another effective way to achieve a good quality of sleep every night is to practice good sleeping habits regularly. Don't use mobile phones and portable computers at night especially while preparing to sleep.

The light that comes from the screen of the electronic devices that were stated has strong impact to the ability of a person to sleep easily at night. Don't eat several amounts of food at night and avoid eating midnight snacks for all these things have negative effects to the ability of a person to achieve good quality of nightly sleep as well.

Learn how to relax while preparing to sleep. Remember, people can't afford to be restless and afraid of something while preparing to sleep. Try to learn how to relax an hour before bedtime for it can also help in providing a human body with a rejuvenating sleep during evening hours.

Most people tend to disregard the importance and the significance of proper sleep patterns. Therefore there is a need to reeducate people of this very important element which is so impactful on the daily functions of anyone.

As sleep is an essential part of a normal and healthy growing individual it should be regarded with some respect. Sleep helps the body to rejuvenate adequately, so that the daily challenges will be better handled.

However at this point it is not completely known how the actual sleep state can be accurately and precisely explained in it's physiologically phenomenon state.

Though thought to be a rather passive state of being it is now know to have a very dynamic process where is brain does not at anytime really shut down complete and instead does perform several unseeing functions within this state, thus it dominant importance.

Basically sleep states can be categorized into different stages such as NREM which is non rapid eye movement and REM which is rapid eye movement.

This then can be broken down even further into other connective categories. It is interesting to note that the sleep cycle experiences several stages in succession over and over again throughout one sleep session and this could take up to about an hour and a half each time. Ideally one should always try to get some level of deep sleep whenever possible through the sleep exercise as this will ensure a better and more refreshed state upon awakening.

Some more detrimental effects of lack of sleep have been documented as having a weaker immune system, lower while blood cell count, decrease in the release of growth hormones, heart rate variability and a host of other problems.

Chapter 2- How to Attain a Rejuvenating Sleep at Night

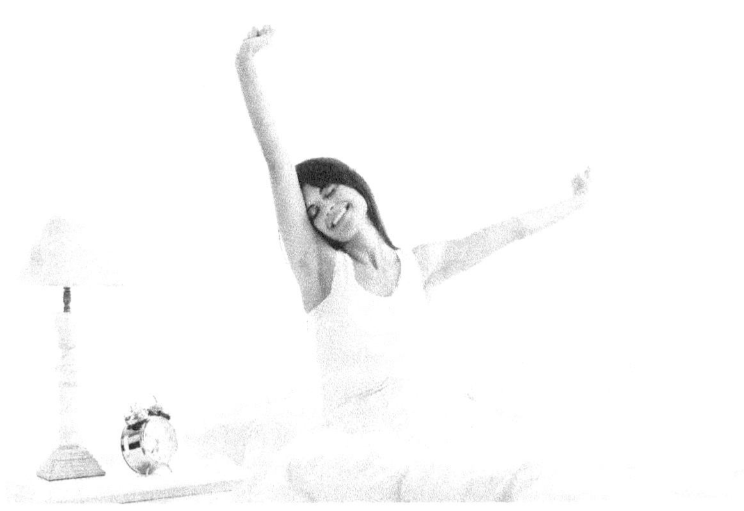

Time management plays an important role in the process of providing a person with a rejuvenating sleep every night. It's one of the most significant factors that can really help a person to sleep for almost eight hours during evening hours while aiming to have a good quality of sleep. Time management usually allows a person to manage a set of activities more effectively during day hours. It can help a person to accomplish a task faster and more efficiently from time to time.

Proper time management can always provide a person with a chance to attain a good quality of sleep every night since it works excellently in the process of preventing stressful moments. It's one of the things that can help a person fight the negative effects of stress more effectively. Time management can also provide a person with a sufficient amount of time for relaxation every night while preparing to sleep and it starts with the ability of a person to keep a regular schedule.

It's really important to keep a regular schedule while aiming to achieve a good quality of nightly sleep every night. This is because it can help a person manage several tasks easily while reserving sufficient amount of time for sleep during evening hours.

Proper time management is very important in the process of organizing a regular schedule. It helps people maximize the use of time in their daily routines. To keep a regular schedule can provide several kinds of amazing benefits in the daily living of a person.

First, it allows a person to save more time in the process of accomplishing a set of tasks. Therefore, it works excellently in the process of increasing the daily productivity of an individual. Second, it's a powerful protection against stress that people can use regularly to keep their daily living happy and highly protected from the negative effects of stress as the time passes by. In other words, it can also help people protect themselves from several kinds of sleep disorders that can be associated with stress and anxiety. But the most interesting benefit that it can offer in the daily living of all people in this world is a good quality of nightly sleep.

Time management allows a person to keep a regular schedule in a very excellent way. An eight-hour sleep during evening hours will never be too difficult for a person to achieve with the help of this amazing strategy. It will not just provide a person with a rejuvenating sleep every night. But also, it can help a person to be more enthusiastic and full of energy during day hours. It also encourages a person to spend more time on recreational activities during day hours instead of having a siesta. Those people who don't want to be victimized by any type of sleep disorder for the rest of their lives should never hesitate to rely on all benefits that proper time management can provide in their daily living.

Sometimes after exhausting all existing tried and true methods of doing things one needs to adjust the mindset to be open to trying new and more innovative ways to solving the sleep deprivation problem. This is especially necessary if the current methods are adding to the stress levels of an already difficult situation.

Here are some suggestions on the changes that can be made in order to create a more easily sought sleep state:

• Taking up a new and slightly more physically demanding exercise regimen. Though exercise has always been an important way of living a healthy lifestyle elevating the requirements of the exercise routine will help to exhaust the body into craving for better rest sessions thus enabling the individual to get good sleep sessions.

• Eating healthier and lighter meals especially before sleep pattern times will also help to create a more conducive body condition so that sleep comes easily and naturally. Eating heavy meals that are also unhealthy in its content will cause such discomfort that the individual will be unable to induce comfortable sleep sessions.

• Being exposed to bright light will also help to keep the brain alert and functioning at its optimum thus exhausting it enough to induce proper sleep patterns when the body feels the need for it. So when working in darker surrounding environments one should always opt to have bright lights enhancing the work area.

• Using the temperature element as an effective tool to induce consistent and successful sleep patterns has been documented as having some level of success. Keeping the temperature at levels which creates a comfortable atmosphere for the individual will eventually allow a more relaxed state to prevail thus inducing sleep.

• Adopting a comfortable posture or body position that is more receptive to creating the comfort zone for a sleep experience is both necessary and effective.

Simply having all the right information and tools will not ensure an individual is well on the way to a good night's sleep. There is a need to put into practice all that has been found or suggested to be helpful in the quest to identify the best and most suitable style for the individual's needs.

The following are some of the methods that are recommended for consideration:

• Forcing sleep is not something that is unachievable. Contrary to popular belief, with the right tools sleep can be successfully induced. Creating the "stage" using limited lightening, playing soft soothing music, getting into comfortable attire, having a comfortable sleeping bed with equally comfortable accessories all help to add to the general inducing exercise.

• Though overly strenuous activities are often discouraged especially closer to desired sleeping times, some form of activity that will cause the individual to be sufficiently tired will be welcomed. This will enhance the body's need for rest and also encourage the individual to seek this rest in the form of sleep.

• Audio distractions are often the reason why people lament about the lack of sleep. Making sure the sleeping environment is free from such distractions will be instrumental in creating a more conducive atmosphere for sleep.

• For most individual who are of the older age group, making a conscious effort to avoid any caffeinated beverage is advised. Even the smallest amount of caffeine content drinks and foods can add to the struggle to gain a good night's sleep.

• Though this method requires some experimental trial exercises, it can be beneficial to know that certain types of foods may induce sleep while other may have the opposite effects like keeping the individual alert. Like caffeine there are other foods that may have this particular reaction when consumed.

Candidly, although it's often mocked, the power nap is among the best tools for busy individuals who have to rely on clearness of thought in order to be the most effectual at what they do. T Basically if virtually all of your work involves thinking and wiggling your fingers on a keyboard, blackboard, or waving a writing utensil over a notepad then this most probably applies to you.

A power nap can cause the difference between a beneficial idea and an eminent idea. It can enhance relationships, both personal and professional; by letting you better center on an individual or group of individuals, their message, and enhance your ability to correctly act upon the newly received info.

A power nap is a curt nap, commonly between 10 and 30 minutes long, assumed in the midst of the day in order to invigorate you for the next part of the day. Power naps are not like steady sleep, so you won't be dazed after taking one. While you may have "dreams", power naps are more related to meditation, where thoughts are permitted to move from the subconscious to the conscious mind and back again without you centering on them. Power naps can be assumed just about anywhere where you are able to fully and honestly relax. The key is that it must be someplace mentally comfy. Physical comfort Is likewise crucial, but without the mental solace, the power nap loses its effect. This is why someplace private is pivotal to the successful power nap.

To begin, find a location where you are able to nap uninterruptedly for at least ten minutes, or for the duration of your power nap. Switch off the lights and, if you wish, put on something restful (or boring) to listen to. You might as well wish to put some sort of an alarm on. Remember to give yourself at least a minute to emerge from the nap process.

Note: One crucial thing to remember is that the longer you sleep, the deeper you'll go, and the more potential you'll be groggy when you awaken.

Audio: If you've had a particularly troubled day, or if you suffer from tinnitus, it might be helpful to have some kind of noise in the background which you are able to both lock on to and push aside at the same time. That's since if you had such a day, then relaxing your mind might take too long, or be almost impossible, unless there's some sound there to focus on. This may be executed with both music and spoken text.

Lighting: This is in reality a bit of a touchy matter. Most individuals urge finding a dark, comfortable place. All the same, that's more of a personal matter. If you're power napping out of doors by a lake then you plainly can't turn the sun off. Also, you might be in an office where you're unable to control the lighting. Or you might not mind the light at all, or even prefer it over dark. Or you may merely be among those folks who don't care either way. Anyway, make certain you know what lighting situation is better for you and find a way to get into that prior to beginning your nap.

When you've discovered a place, make yourself comfy by lying down and loosening your body. It's crucial that you lay facing up, even if you're a side- or stomach-sleeper, as this pose will keep your back in suitable alignment and will make it easier for your body to speedily unwind. Ensure that your shoulders and arms are totally relaxed.

From this spot it's all in your head, literally. The enticement here will be to start thinking of something, anything, actively. Don't! If an idea comes to your mind, that's fine, let it be there, but don't center on it; don't sustain it. Merely let it come and goes.

Concentrate on your breathing. Center on how your nostrils feel when air draws in and out, or how the air feels when it hits the back of your throat. If you're playing something, center on the sound of the instruments or voice, but don't center on the tune, or what's being said. Keep doing that as long as you require. This way, no idea can take root, and your mind will start to unload info faster. It might seem that your mind is now full and that you're considering too much, but remember that you're not thinking about anything, ideas are just passing. Your mind is now discharging information, and this is precisely what you want it to do.

Quickly you should almost feel like you're beginning to dream. You might, in fact, do so. That's o.k... It means you're at ease and your mind is refreshing itself.

If you've an alarm, when it goes off, merely open your eyes and lay there. Your alarm shouldn't be too intrusive. You don't want to frighten yourself out of your nap. Most mobile phones have alarm features which will serve this purpose. Center on your breathing and open your eyes. Feel your body and begin to stretch along. Sit up easy and take it all in. Your mind should be clear now.

Chapter 3- Bedtime Routine to Regulate Your Sleep Naturally

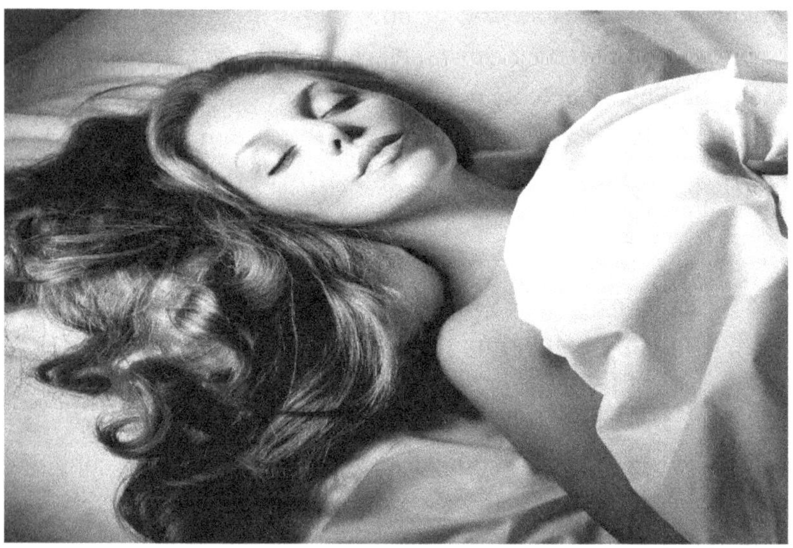

The process of regulating sleep cycles has never been too easy in this world especially to those professional individuals and businessmen who don't have consistent work schedules. This is a huge burden in the daily living of those individuals who want to have a good quality of sleep in their daily living.

There are so many ways to regulate sleep cycles naturally. People don't need to rely on sleeping pills while trying to regulate their sleep cycles more effectively. Some of the new discoveries in field of Science nowadays have proven all individuals in this world can naturally regulate their sleep cycles without spending a lot of effort by changing their sleeping environment positively and controlling their diet more efficiently. Read the remaining parts of this chapter to understand the most effective ways on how to regulate sleep cycles naturally.

Many people have inconsistent schedules due to their job descriptions and nature of work. Such reality makes the process of achieving a good quality of sleep more difficult for almost 50% of the total population in this world. But with the help of Science and modern technology, scientists have successfully discovered the most effective ways on how to naturally regulate sleep cycles when needed.

There are two steps to follow while aiming to regular sleep cycles naturally. Sleeping pills are not needed in the process of completing all these steps.

First, try to create a sleeping environment that's always inaccessible for light. Construct a bedroom in an area that's always protected from sunlight and provide its windows with curtains. Make sure that its location is not too close in places where environmental noises are always available like public highways/streets and playgrounds. Good sleeping environment is one of the most effective strategies that people can use to regulate their sleep cycles naturally in accordance to the sudden changes in their schedules. But this is not enough in providing good quality of sleep for those individuals who don't have consistent schedules. The second step on how to naturally regulate sleep cycles is to have a quick change in diet.

Don't eat for almost 16 hours while preparing for a new change in sleep schedule. This is the most important strategy that a person has to execute while aiming to regulate sleep cycles naturally. It can help people adapt to new changes in their sleep schedules more effectively without relying on all benefits that sleeping pills can offer. These steps on how to regulate sleep cycles naturally are 100% safe and effective. Remember these steps always while aiming to learn the most effective ways on how to naturally regulate sleep cycles. It's unwise to rely on sleeping pills since these products contain synthetic ingredients that can cause harmful side effects on a human body.

A relaxing bedtime routine is always important in the process of providing a person with good quality of sleep every night. It's something that can help a person fall asleep easily during evening hours without taking a sleeping pill that's very harmful and full of synthetic ingredients. A comprehensive knowledge on how to relax more effectively before bedtime is a great advantage for those people who want to have an excellent bedtime routine in their daily living. Excellent bedtime routine is one of the things that can help a person to sleep more comfortably during evening hours.

Several individuals in the different parts of the globe have already proven that relaxing bedtime routine works excellently in the process of providing an individual with a rejuvenating sleep every day. This is because it encourages a person to relax and rest more comfortably while preparing to sleep. It's something that can relieve all negative effects of stress and tiredness in a human body in a very efficient way. It will never fail the expectations of those individuals who always want to be protected from the negative effects of sleep disorders like insomnia for the rest of their lives. Some people consider it the most effective solution to all problems of those individuals who always suffer from sleepless nights.

In this chapter, people will learn the most effective ways on how to achieve a relaxing bedtime routine.

The process of creating a relaxing bedtime routine takes a lot of time and effort. A person who really wants to have a good quality of sleep every day should never give up in the completion of all its standard requirements. One of the most important things that a person has to accomplish while aiming to understand the real meaning of a relaxing bedtime routine is a regular or fixed schedule. There's a need to master the most effective tips on proper time management while aiming to create an excellent bedtime routine.

Remember, proper time management allows a person to accomplish several tasks faster and most efficiently every day. It's something that can provide an individual with a sufficient amount of time for relaxation and sleep during evening hours. A person who wants to have a good quality of sleep every night should perform a relaxing activity an hour before bedtime. One good example of a relaxing activity that a person can perform while preparing to sleep is to lie on a bed for several minutes while thinking of happy moments in life.

Turn off the lights and don't use any type of electronic gadget at this stage. Play a relaxing music with slow tempo and wonderful melody while relaxing and then turn off the player when it's already time to sleep. Don't forget to organize an excellent bedtime schedule while aiming to achieve the best benefits that a relaxing bedtime routine can provide to all people in this world who deserve to be protected from the negative effects of restlessness, irritability, sleeplessness and serious medical conditions for the rest of their lives.

The physical component calls for the tensing and relaxing of muscle groups over the arms, legs, face, stomach and chest. With the eyes shut and in a successive pattern, a tension in a given muscle group is purposefully caused for approximately ten seconds and then discharged for twenty seconds before going along with the next muscle group.

The mental component centers on the difference between the feelings of the tension and relaxation. As the eyes are shut, one is impelled to center on the sensation of tension and relaxation. In persons with anxiousness, the mind often thinks "I don't know if this will work" or "Am I experiencing it yet." If such is the case, the person is told to simply center on the feelings of the tensed up muscle. Because of the feelings of warmth and weightiness are felt in the relaxed muscle after it's tensed up, a mental relaxation is experienced as a result.

1. Once you have found a quiet place and a few free minutes to rehearse progressive muscle relaxation, sit down or lie down and make yourself easy.

2. Start out by tensing up all the muscles in your face. Constitute a tight grimace, shut your eyes as tightly as conceivable, clinch your teeth, even move your ears up if you are able to. Carry on this part for the count of 8 as you breathe in.

3. Now breathe out and loosen up entirely. Let your face go totally loose, as if you were sleeping. Feel the tautness ooze from your facial muscles, and delight in the feeling.

4. Following, wholly tense up your neck and shoulders, once again breathing in and counting to 8. Then breathe out and loosen up.

5. Carry on down your body, duplicating the routine with the following muscle groups:

• Chest

• Stomach

• Total right arm

• Right forearm and hand (establishing a fist)

• Right hand

• Total left arm

• Left forearm and hand (once again, establishing a fist)

- Left hand

- Buttocks

- Total right leg

- Lower right leg and foot

- Right foot

- Total left leg

- Lower left leg and foot

- Left foot

6. For the abbreviated variation, this sets in just 4 chief muscle groups:

- Face

- Neck, shoulders and arms

- Stomach and chest

- Buttocks, legs and feet

Rapidly centering on each group one after the other, with rehearsal you are able to relax your body like, liquefied relaxation" poured out on your head and it flowed down and totally covered you. You are able to use progressive muscle relaxation to rapidly de-stress any time as well as to get ready your body for a good night sleep.

Upon being studied it was found that practices of this technique could slow their breathing by twenty-five percent, diminish their oxygen consumption by seventeen percent, lower their blood pressure, and slow down their pulse rate.

In order to make the technique more approachable and scientific, researchers removed the Eastern religious factor and condensed the basic strategy of Transcendental Meditation, which is said to be a component of every major religious tradition or meditative pattern—the repeating of a word, sound, prayer, or phrasal idiom to the exclusion of other thinking.

Nowadays, this technique helps individuals manage the negative effects of stress and reduce stress-related symptoms as well as improve their sleep.

How to accomplish the strategy:

1. Discover a calm and quiet place and sit down in a comfy position. Attempt to loosen up all your muscles.

2. Shut your eyes.

3. Select a word, phrase, or prayer to center on that has particular meaning to you, is securely rooted in your belief system, or makes you feel at peace a few examples are "one", "serenity", "I am with you Lord", "I am one with the universe", or even a word like "thankful".

4. Take a breath slowly and naturally. Breathe in through your nose and hesitate for a couple of seconds. Breathe out through your mouth, once again hesitating for a couple of seconds. Wordlessly say your focus word, phrase, or prayer as you breathe out.

5. Do not concern yourself about how well you are doing and do not feel badly if thoughts or feelings trespass in your mind. Merely say to yourself "Oh well" and go back to your repeating.

6. When the time comes to the end, remain aware of your breathing but sit down quietly. Getting aware of where you are, slowly open up your eyes and rise bit by bit.

This strategy is generally practiced for ten to twenty minutes per day, or at the least 3 to 4 times a week.

If you have to keep track of the time, try utilizing an alarm or timer set on the smallest volume, so you don't have to keep viewing your watch or clock.

Stress can cause severe wellness problems and, in extreme cases, can induce death. While stress management techniques have been shown to have a positive effect on reducing stress and bettering sleep, they're for guidance only, and readers should take the advice of fittingly qualified health care providers if they have any concerns over stress-related illnesses or if stress is causing significant or persistent unhappiness and loss of sleep.

Chapter 4- Importance of Good Quality Sleep in Your Daily Living

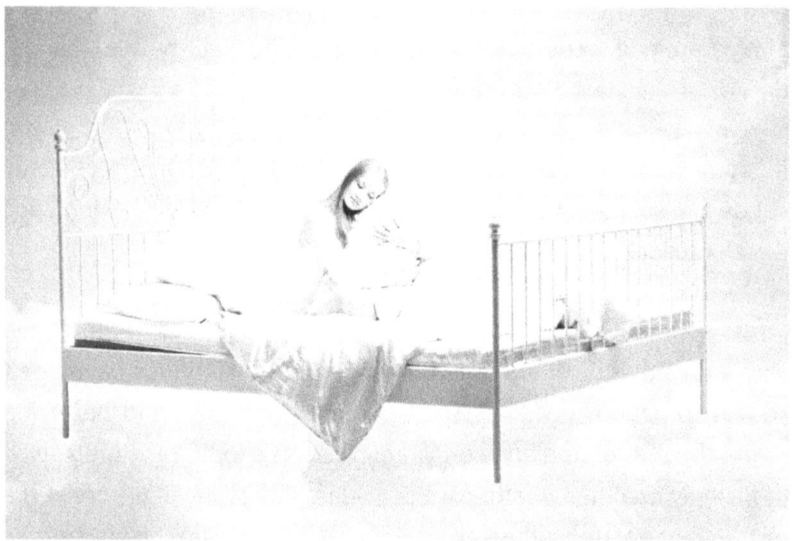

Many people in this world believe that better living starts with good sleeping habits. Scientific studies have proven that good quality of sleep can help people stay strong and full of energy in their daily living.

Such things play an important role in the process of enhancing the overall status of an individual. People can leave happily for the rest of their lives if all of them will never fail to achieve all requirements that are necessary in achieving a good quality of sleep. Good sleeping habits were proven effective when it comes to the process of preserving the good health of a person who deserves to live longer in this world.

Healthy diet and regular exercise are not sufficient when it comes to the process of providing a person with a better way of living. Such things are still useless if a good quality of sleep is not available in the daily living of a person. Lack of good quality of sleep can make a person weak and prone to several kinds of serious medical conditions as the time passes by. Studies have also proven that poor quality of nightly sleep can make a person fat and prone to the negative effects of obesity.

Good quality of sleep is one of the things that can really provide a person with s better way of living in this world as the time passes by. It allows a human body to be rejuvenated in a very natural way. In addition to that, it keeps a person protected from several kinds of harmful sleep disorders that are not too easy to treat and can destroy the excellent health status of an individual in an instant when not treated properly. There's no need to rely on sleeping pills while trying to start a better way of living with good quality of sleep. This is because it's too easy to achieve with good sleeping habits and a relaxing bedtime routine.

Good sleeping habits usually encourage a person to sleep for almost eight hours every day. It can prevent the production of harmful toxins in the brain and other parts of the body of a person when regularly executed. It's more reliable and efficient than dietary supplements, sleeping pills and other types of synthetic medicines that are containing processed ingredients. Executing good sleeping habits or routine regularly is the safest and most effective way of improving the overall quality of the lifestyle of an individual. Such things have an amazing ability to keep a person active and reliable during day hours. Good quality of sleep is something that can help an individual to become more productive and always protected from several kinds of serious medical conditions at all times.

Chapter 5- Using Food & Aromatherapy to Sleep Better

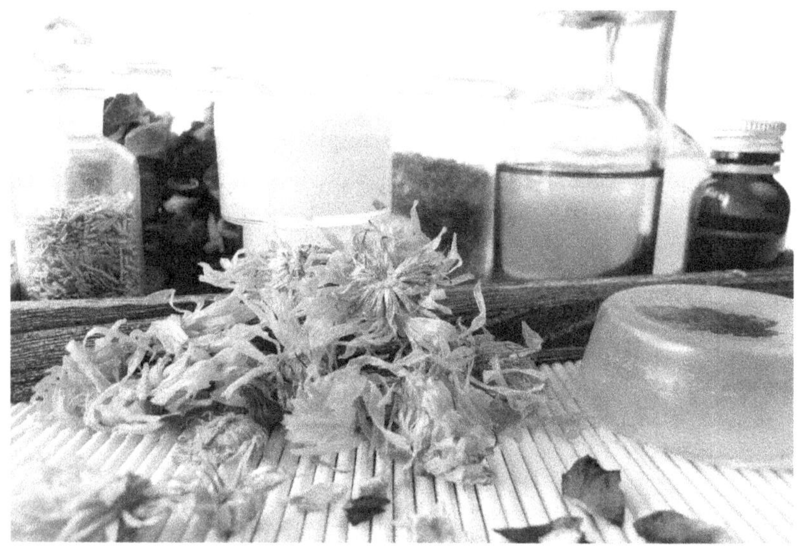

There are Sleep inducing foods or foods high in tryptophan are beneficial sleep aids. Prior to hitting the sack, try one or more of the following foods to assist you in sleep. The basic denominator in these foods is that they contain tryptophan which has been demonstrated to assist sleep:

- Sesame seeds

- Spirolina

- Spinach

- Bananas

- Figs

- Dates

- Soy

- Turkey

- Silken Tofu

Turkey

Get a mental picture of granddad last Thanksgiving Day: at rest on the couch, head back, belt open -and it was only six p.m. It's not his 80 years it's the turkey. Turkey holds tryptophan, an aminoalkanoic acid that turns to the sleep - advancing neurotransmitter serotonin. To feel the turkey sleep enhancer, try eating a turkey sandwich 60 minutes before bedtime.

Warm milk

Equivalent to turkey, milk bears tryptophan, and the calcium and magnesium in milk assist and enhance the transition of tryptophan to serotonin. As for whether there's any reality to the old story about warm milk's slumber - causing powers, there is no study out yet.

It is believe for a long time that warming the milk makes the tryptophan more bio available to the body. However no one has ever executed a clinical study on warm milk vs. cold milk. If the idea of warm milk makes you feel all warm and fuzzy inside, apply it. If it makes you want to gag, gulp it cold. Either direction, try out a glass an hour prior to bedtime.

Prevent these foods prior to bedtime as they've been demonstrated to interrupt sleep patterns:

- Intoxicants

- Sugar

- Sauerkraut

- Cocoa

● Caffeine

● Teas & herbaceous plants

A different option to prescription slumber aids are teas made from these herbaceous plants which have shown to be good as a natural slumber aid

● Nepeta cataria

● Hops

● Valerian root (which is in liquid or capsule forms)

● Passionflower vine (brew with chamomile)

● Skullcap

● Chamaemelum nobilis

Good vitamin supplementations

In addition to sound foods, there are measures of nutritional supplements that may also help remedy sleeplessness. Calcium has long been acclaimed as a natural slumber aid. Think of the advice to drink a warm cup of milk to get better sleep. You are able to get better results by taking 1000 mg of Calcium lactate, or 1500-2000 mg calcium chelate. If having calcium chelate, it is suggested to take it in split up doses.

Try 1000 mg of Magnesium instead of prescription slumber aids. These supplementations are best taken after meals and at bedtime

Likewise helpful to get more beneficial slumber is B complex plus extra pantothen; Inositol, and B6. Always observe the label recommendations.

This is a fantastic slumber aid! While L-theanine doesn't bring on sleep it does calm the "engaged mind" and does bring on alpha rhythm activity in the brain. (It's among the ingredients listed in Melissa, an all natural slumber aid.) This free form aminoalkanoic acid, gained from green tea, quiets and relaxes without side effects.

Additional conditions to get more beneficial slumber.

• A different cause of insomnia may include copper and iron inadequacies in adult females. A hair analysis ought to be done to ascertain if such inadequacies are present.

• Fresh air, melatonin, decompressing with a book, calming music, and a regular schedule are likewise effectual natural slumber aids.

• Yoga and other loosening techniques help clear the mind and abbreviate stress, preparing the body for sleep.

• Make sure to visit your physician to eliminate any rudimentary physical condition that might preclude you from sleeping.

In aromatherapy, the essential oils are utilized topically instead of being taken internally. The essential oils are said to perk up an area of the brain, known as the limbic system that commands mood and emotion. Firm scientific backing for aromatherapy is deficient, but there's info, without doubt, that many individuals find it a soothing complement to other self-help measures to ease stress, promote relaxation behavior, and aid in sleep as part of their bedtime readings. So you might prefer to give it a try.

To assist in restoring restful slumber, you are able to try utilizing essential oils one by one or in combination. The essential oils are typically available at health food stores, while these days many pharmacies as well carry a variety of the oils. The most normally advocated oil for promoting sleep is lavender, but there are a lot of others that may have a soothing effect.

Try out adding a couple of drops of essential oil to warm water for an unwinding bath or footbath, or spray the oil onto a hankie or small pillow. You are able to as well utilize a few drops to a heat diffuser near your bed to disperse the scent through the room or use a particularly made ring that can be placed on the electric-light bulb of a bedside lamp; the heat of the bulb circulates the scent.

You may as well prefer to try blending the relaxing benefits of aromatherapy and massage by making your own scented massage oil. Dilute one to 3 drops of essential oil per teaspoonful of unscented carrier oil, like almond or grape-seed oil. (Do not utilize undiluted essential oil by placing directly on to your skin.) Since some individuals are more sensitive to the oils than other people, begin with the littlest amount, and experiment till you determine the combination that works best for you.

Research is beginning to confirm lavender's tranquilizing qualities. It's been discovered to lengthen total sleep time, step-up deep sleep, and make individuals feel reinvigorated. It seems to work better for adult females, maybe because women tend to have a more intense olfactory modality.

The beneficial thing about lavender is that it starts to work quickly. Once again try placing a lavender sachet under your pillow or place one to two drops of lavender essential oil in a hankie. Or add several drops of lavender oil to a bath -- the drop in body temperature after a warm bath as well assists with better sleep.

You can as well make a sweet smelling sleep pillow.

Having a pleasant scent filling up your nostrils when you get into bed might help you drop off to dreamland. A perfumed pillow is one way to produce this effect. To create a scented pillow, you are able to, naturally, spray a little of essential oil onto your regular pillow. But you are able to as well create an herb-filled sleep pillow by mixing aromatic herbs and sewing them into a small piece of soft fabric. You'll want the pillow to be modest and flat, so you are able to slip it into your regular pillow slip, on top of your regular pillow. Here's a sweet but powerful mixture for an herbal pillow:

- 4 parts dried out lavender leaves

- 2 parts dried out hops

- 2 parts dried out rose petals

- 1 part dried out chamomile

- 1 part dried out lemon balm

The herbs finally lose their scent and ought to be replaced after about nine to twelve months.

Chapter 6- Negative Results of Poor Sleeping

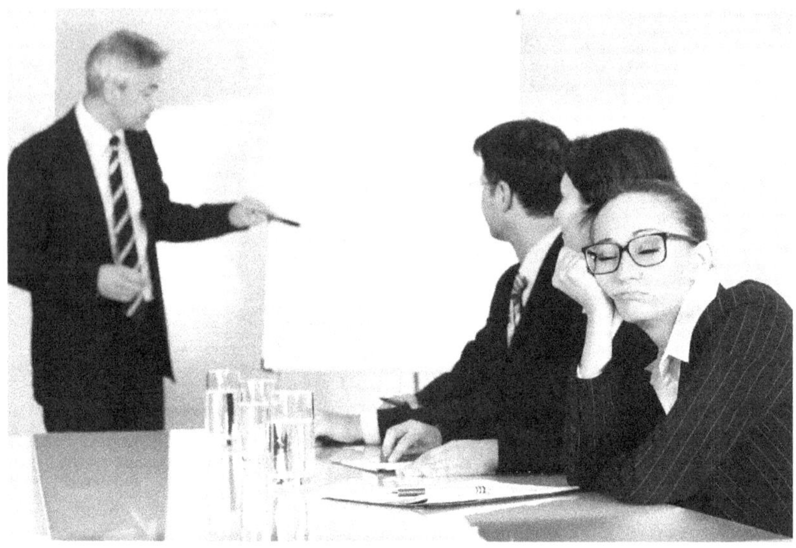

Failing to give due importance to this very significant part of the human existence can and will results in some very negative results. The following are just some negative repercussions for not taking the importance of good sleeping patterns into consideration:

• Poor quality and quantity of work may become evident when there is a general lack of sleep. This will cause the individual to have lack of concentration and thus produce unacceptable work. Unnecessary mistakes and substandard work will then contribute to even bigger problems especially when the said work is a contributing part of an overall team effort. Colleagues will then begin to question the relevance of having such an individual as a team member and this may eventually lead to one's job being in jeopardy.

• Becoming short tempered and irritable is also another negative trait that will be prevalent when there is lack of sleep. This can then lead to relationship problems. If left unchecked this negative behavior may spill into other aspects of the individual's life causing damage along the way that may not be salvaged.

• Making rash decisions or wrong decisions is also a byproduct of not having enough sleep as the brain in unable to function at its optimum. Here too some of these decisions may cause such negative repercussions that it may be difficult if not impossible to rectify.

• Once, erratic sleep patterns have become the norm it may be very difficult to reestablish better and more manageable sleep routines.

You might never have blundered so dramatically, but the odds are you're not getting the 7 to 8 hours of nightly shuteye experts agree you require. While a few high-achieving entrepreneurs boast of taking minimal, research demonstrates that our sleep needs are astonishingly consistent. If you fail to get at least 7 nightly hours, you're likely operating at a cognitive disadvantage.

And your health and your business might be paying the price. Business owners seem to share a hefty ambivalence toward sleep, both craving and ostracizing it. That's particularly true in this bad economy - a recent poll found that small-business owners are working longer, thanks to the decline - and during a startup stage.

So what? You enquire. Aren't you more productive when you work eighteen hour days? Can't you just shore up your droopy eyelids by downing yet another cup of coffee?

Unfortunately, no new scientific research demonstrates that going without enough sleep for more than an occasional day or two can play havoc on your wellness, memory, concentration, temper, and ability to arrive at decisions - even if you believe you're doing all right.

Sleeping Secrets

If you require a good reason to begin sacking out earlier or sleeping later, here it is. It turns out that far from being a time waster, sleep makes you fitter, smarter, and a more beneficial leader - and might even yield great thoughts for growing your business.

The evidence that sleep matters is incontrovertible and perpetually growing. Let's begin with a freshly discovered link between sleep loss and serious sicknesses like diabetes and cancer. A 2008 scientific research at the University of Chicago's school of medicine kept young, healthy volunteers alert for all but 4 hours a night for 6 nights running. The resultant: The levels of subjects' hormones shifted - particularly a hormone called leptin that bears on appetite. They got ravenously hungry, gulping down pizza and ice cream long after they'd have felt full generally, and their blood glucose shot up to pre-diabetic levels - a menacing result after less than one week of poor sleep.

Other analyses repeat those results so regularly that researchers now trust that not getting enough sleep is a lead cause of obesity and diabetes, both of which are on the rise across the country. At the same time, the WHO has accumulated data from around the Earth showing that sleep loss depresses the immune system, to the point where WHO is thinking about labeling chronic sleep loss a carcinogen, comparable to tobacco and asbestos.

If you've ever been so tired out that you had to reread the same paragraph several times to grip its meaning and soon blanked out what you read, you already know what sleep investigators have lately demonstrated about the effects of too little sack time on productivity.

One experiment at a school of medicine kept subjects up until four A.M., woke them at eight A.M., and then fed them a series of tests designed to measure memory, vigilance, and the ability to react quickly to fresh data. The researchers were startled to find that subjects' mental acuity slumped markedly after just one night and kept falling with each successive night of 4 hours' sleep. Even more distressing: The study's volunteers were incognizant of their deterioration. One woman, so tired that she could barely say her name, was all the same sure she was able to drive home.

Regardless how much you believe you're achieving when you pull an all-nighter, it's likely to a lesser degree than what you could accomplish if you got some sleep then returned to work. Studies gave volunteers a list of words to memorize and then were kept alert for twenty-four hours, their power to recall the words fell by forty%. Memory betters during sleep, so that if you get a full 7 or 8 hours sleep tonight, your recall of all that happened today will be twenty% to thirty% sharper than it is directly after the day's events happen. No one is for certain yet why this is so.

For entrepreneurs, the finest reason to get enough shuteye might be to avoid making dense, costly decisions. A sleep researcher recently gave 3 groups of subjects the same pieces of data. Those who walked off and spent at least 7 of the next 12 hours sleeping were able to brand broader and more lucid connections than those who didn't get much (or any) sleep or those who attempted to analyze the data right away.

A lot of successful CEOs discuss having good instincts. I'd argue that all they're doing is permitting them at least twelve hours to marinate the data they absorb - and if those twelve hours include some sleep, they get even finer results.

CHAPTER 7- NEGATIVE EFFECT OF STRESS AND TENSION

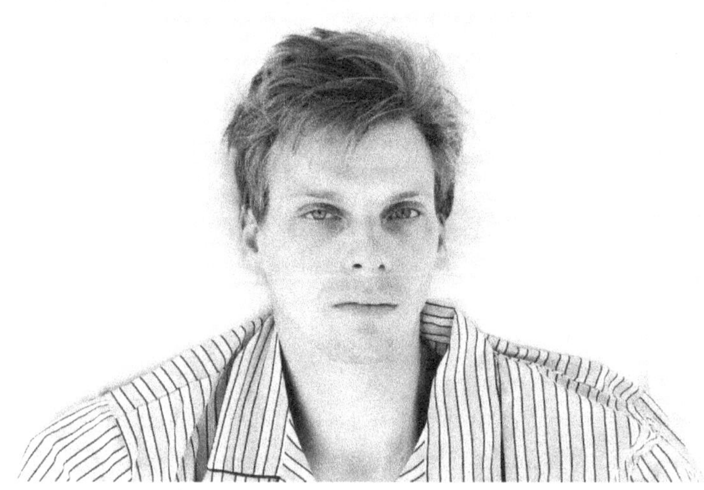

Stress and tension are common types of medical conditions that can make the daily living of a person miserable and sad. These medical conditions can be treated. But it takes a lot of time to remove all its negative effects in the daily living of a person who doesn't know how to achieve a good quality of sleep as the time passes by.

One of the most effective treatments that people can use to fight and eliminate the negative effects of stress and tension in their daily living is to rely on all benefits that excellent bedtime routine can offer.

Relaxing bedtime routine is something that can help a person to relax and stay free from the negative effects of tiredness while preparing to sleep. Aside from that, good quality of sleep can provide a person with a better way of living since it plays an important role in balancing the most important growth hormones in a human body. It will never fail the expectations of those individuals who want to grow healthier and strong as the time passes by regardless of the presence of tough tasks and responsibilities that are meant to be completed in their daily living.

Stress and tension will never be able to survive in the amazing healing benefits that good quality of sleep can provide in a human body. Remember, it helps a human body to be rejuvenated naturally every morning. It can also preserve the excellent status of the mental health of a person as the time passes by.

But a person doesn't need to sleep for more than eight hours every night while aiming to fight the negative effects of stress and tension more efficiently.

This is because too much sleep can make all negative effects of stress and tension in a human body worst and more difficult to treat. Excessive sleep is not good for those people who want to be protected from the negative effect of chronic diseases as well.

Many people in this world believe that synthetic medicine is the only thing that can help a patient to fight the negative effects of stress and tension more effectively. But such belief is a big mistake.

This is because synthetic medicines are not really safe and effective to use in the process of treating a patient who suffers from stress and tension. Such type of medicines have harmful side effects that can make all things more dangerous when it comes to the process of eliminating the negative effects of medical conditions that were stated in the body of a patient.

Having good sleeping habits is one of the most effective ways on how to fight stress and tension naturally. Those people who don't know how to improve their sleeping habits will never be able to protect themselves from the different kinds of sleep disorders that stress and tension might create in their health status. Remember, stressful moments and tension are included in the list of medical conditions that can also affect the ability of an individual to fall asleep faster during evening hours.

Getting back to sleep during evening hours will never be too difficult to execute for those individuals who have relaxing bedtime routine at all times. One of the things that can affect the ability of an individual to get back to sleep easily is a sleep disorder. But this problem won't be able to affect the daily living of a person who possesses good sleeping habits that are really necessary in the process of creating an excellent bedtime routine. In this chapter, the most effective ways on how to get back to sleep easily will be enumerated for the benefit of those individuals who really want to be happy and always protected from several kinds of serious medical conditions for the rest of their lives.

There are so many ways to get back to sleep easily during evening hours while aiming for a good quality of sleep. Such things have been proven effective when it comes to the process of providing a person with a rejuvenating sleep regardless of the different types of disturbances that may occur in their sleeping environment from time to time. There's no need to rely on sleeping pills and massage therapies while aiming to get back to sleep faster during evening hours. A person's determination and willingness to sleep better during evening hours is already enough in the process of mastering the most effective ways on how to get back to sleep easily.

Many people in this world suffer from serious medical conditions and stress from time to time even though their regular diet is good. Such individuals are those who don't have good quality of nightly sleep most of the time. Good quality of sleep is always important in the process of improving the overall health status of a person. It works excellently in the process of rejuvenating a human body as well. But it's not too easy to achieve a good quality of nightly sleep during evening hours. In fact, there are so many sleep requirements to prepare while aiming to achieve the best benefits that it can provide.

One of the most effective steps than can be performed to get back to sleep easily during evening hours is to learn how to relax. A relaxing bedtime routine is always significant in getting back to sleep easily. It encourages a person to spend an hour on relaxing activities while preparing to sleep. One good example of relaxing activity that a person can perform to get back to sleep faster is to listen into a wonderful music that has a slow tempo and relaxing melody while lying on a bed. To stay quiet and free from the negative effects of worrying can also help a person to get back to sleep faster during evening hours without spending a lot of effort.

The easiest way to get back to sleep easily during evening hours is to perform non-stimulating activities while preparing to sleep. Like for example is to avoid using backlight devices and electronic gadgets while resting.

CHAPTER 8- WHEN TO SEEK HELP & SUPPORT GROUPS

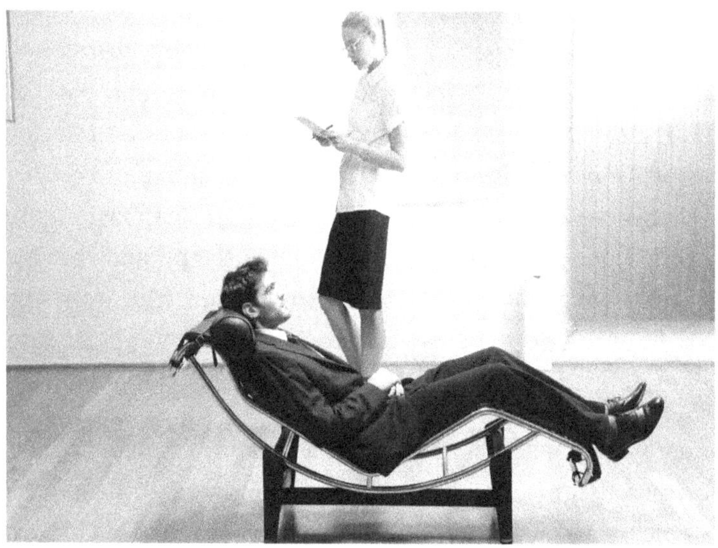

For a lot of people today sleep is something that is always last to be considered.

Generally especially the younger generation think that sleep is not really important and definitely a waste of their precious time.

However it should be noted that generally when such individuals do attempt to get some sleep it is often very difficult to wake them up.

However the importance of sleep should not be discounted and working out the elements that are causing the lack of sleep or the inability to get proper sleep would be most beneficial.

Ironically the huge number of individuals do experience some form of sleep deprivation and its negative effects fairly often though, there are times when this comes about without the actual realization of its occurrence.

Taking the time and effort to find out if this phenomenon is occurring randomly in one's life with or without significant impact being caused is worth the trouble so that the situation can be addressed and rectified.

Some may explain it as sleep homeostasis which generally implies that the more sleep an individual is able to experience the less likelihood of the individual nodding off to sleep at the slightest opportunity and the more there is loss of sleep the more significant the need to sleep will be.

There are several possibilities why this may occur and some of them are too many distractions, non conducive environment, high stress levels, too many things that need immediate attention and the list is never ending.

Indentifying some of the more popular possibilities that are causing the lack of sleep will help the individual the focus on rectifying the situation or at the very least seeking suitable solution that will help ease the inability for sleep opportunities. When the opportunity has been given to identify the reason for the sleep deprivation than besides finding solutions the individual must also resolve not to "fall back" into the same negative situation at a later stage.

There are several types of goal setting exercises that can be adopted to suit the need of sleeping. These goals will vary greatly from one person to another, so there is a need to define what your goals are as an individual within the realm of sleep.

When this is successfully done then the identification of the necessary elements that will produce the desired results can then be designed.

Family goals are a very powerful way to build trust, communication, togetherness and many other positive elements. It's also a good way to encouraging children to learn how to set goals within their own little worlds. Here are some recommendations that can be followed in the pursuit to identifying and setting goals:

• The exercise of setting goals should be done with the participation of every family member. This participation should be active rather than passive and age should not be a deterrent. Younger children can sometimes be surprisingly insightful and can come up with very workable solutions to a particular goal.

• Limiting the amount of goals the family has to work with is also advised. When there is too much going on, there will be very little concentrated focus on actually making a success of the goal and its eventual positive results.

• Identifying and setting the goals should not be limited to any particular time of the year or phase in a family member's life. These exercises should be done if and when necessary and is a spontaneous fashion to ensure there is not threatening feelings arising.

• Setting up an incentive plan within the goal setting exercise will also encourage maximum participation and results of all the family members.

• Sometimes it may be necessary to set a time frame for the intended goals set. This is to ensure some results can be forthcoming rather that constant procrastination.

Good quality of nightly sleep is one of the things that can really help a person to stay healthy and protected from the negative effects of serious medical conditions and harmful diseases as the time goes by. However, it will never be too easy to achieve for those individuals who always find it difficult to fall asleep faster during evening hours. There are so many factors that can affect the ability of a person to sleep faster every night. A sleep disorder is an example of factors that can affect the ability of a person to sleep easily every day.

Sleep disorders can be treated. There are so many kinds of synthetic medicines in the field of healthcare industry that people can use to fight the negative effects sleep disorders more effectively. But those individuals who really want to discover the safest ways to treat or eliminate sleep disorders should never hesitate to consult a doctor as soon as possible. This is because a physician who specializes in various types of medicines and therapies for sleep disorders is the only type of healthcare agent that can provide a person with comprehensive knowledge on how to treat sleep disorders naturally with the use of relaxing sleep habits.

Those people who suffer from insomnia and other types of sleep disorders should ask for the professional assistance that a physician can provide as soon as possible. This is because sleep disorders are very dangerous and can also affect the health status of an individual unnoticeably as the time passes by.

Sleep disorders are not good for the health of all people in this world. The poor quality of sleep that these disorders can provide in the daily living of an individual causes several kinds of harmful medical conditions that can shorten the life of a person unnoticeably.

Studies have proven that lack of rejuvenating sleep is one of the main reasons why many people in this world suffer from the negative effects of serious medical conditions like cancer and heart diseases as the time passes by.

Those people who believe that the daily quality of their sleep is not good enough to make them strong and healthier every day should never hesitate to consult a doctor as soon as possible for it's the only type of professional individual who can guide them in improving their sleeping habits.

A doctor may also recommend a certain type of synthetic medicine to those individuals who suffered from a certain type of sleep disorder for several months to help them get back to sleep faster during evening hours. Physicians can also share some tips and advice to those individuals who want provide themselves with relaxing bedtime routine.

ABOUT THE AUTHOR

Emil McAdams have written various books on different areas of health because he's been an avid reader of many types of health books. He's been interested in health books for countless years so decided to write on each subject what he have found out from all the other books and condensed them into one easy to read book in laymen's terms to make it easier for people to understand and thus implement into their daily lives.